3/10/22?

D1473424

THE ESSENTIAL

DREAM

JOURNAL

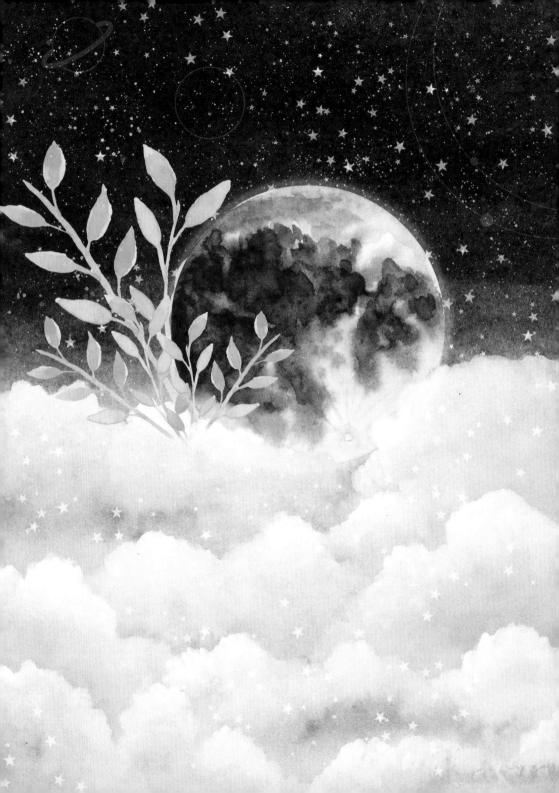

THE ESSENTIAL

DREAM

JOURNAL

Record & Interpret the Hidden
Meanings in Your Dreams

ROCK
POINT
QUARTOKNOWS.COM
NEW YORK, NY

Introduction

Shakespeare wrote, "We are such stuff as dreams are made on." Every part of your dreams is intrinsically made up of your *self*. The tiniest details in your dreams correspond to coded messages your brain is trying to send you. These everyday impressions of a house, a car, your second cousin twice removed, all have a meaning—if only you know how to translate it to your conscious mind.

Sleep is important to every conscious creature, and not just sleep, but the deep REM sleep that brings about your dreams. Rats who are deprived of this precious type of sleep will often forgo normal rat behavior such as burrowing and grooming. If we translate this to our human bodies, our dreams are where our subconscious runs obscure scenarios to help us cope with our waking life. By taking a close look at your dreams, you can decipher the subtle secrets of your subconscious mind.

Our dreams are enigmatic and hard to pin down (as dreams are supposed to be), but with this guide and journal you'll be better equipped to interpret the signs and symbols that frequently recur, courtesy of your subconscious.

Dreams often reflect some of the emotions, obstacles, and behaviors that we exhibit in our actual lives. Sometimes, we may interpret our dreams to have spiritual meanings, especially if we dream of a deceased loved one trying to communicate with us. There are many dream interpretations to help guide us through our mind's messages.

One of the most important aspects of understanding dreams—regardless of your interpretation methods—is journaling. Writing down dreams while they are still fresh in your mind is one of the few habits all experts on the subject absolutely agree is worthwhile; therefore, we have created this journal, where you can record your dreams for later examination.

Reflect back to previous dreams or record new ones, find the connections between recurring dreams, and discover common themes. Translate what your mind is trying to tell you to help guide you in your daily life.

Sources of Dreams

There are no definitive rules for where our dreams come from, but here are some of the most frequent stimuli:

1. Dreams tend to reflect impressions of the few days preceding.

2. Recent and significant experiences are united by the dream into a whole.

3. Dreams choose their imagery according to principles other than those of our waking memory. Our subconscious recalls not what is essential and important, but what is subordinate and disregarded.

4. The earliest memories of our childhood bring light and detail into our current situation.

5. Physical sensations that your sleeping body is experiencing can influence your dreaming.

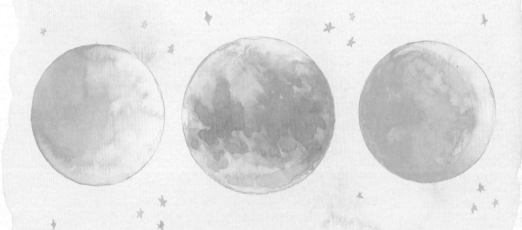

Using This Journal

This is a tool for you to jot down the moving pieces of your hidden thoughts and to track their activity over a long period of time. For best results, try to use this journal daily, even if you can only recall general themes, feelings, and vague impressions of characters. The daily routine of recording your dreams will help keep the door to your subconscious open for longer each time.

Prompts for a slew of different important imagery and themes will help guide you through dream interpretation. Take your time, but don't force the dream into these boxes if they don't fit. The things that are absent from your dreams are just as important as the imagery that fills them. For example, you may find a nightly trend that your dreams are bizarrely devoid of location. This could mean that you are feeling lost, unmoored, and in need of grounding.

After you've recorded the key points of your dream, refer to this first section for common symbols and themes to see if there are any traditional interpretations. People have been recording their dreams for many years and taking their wisdom into account will help you progress in your own interpretations. However, all the wisdom in the world doesn't mean much if it doesn't resonate with you. These rules for dream interpretation are far from stringent. If at any point you think that the language of these symbols is not the language of your mind, use your intuition to try to come up with your own ways to communicate.

Finally, continue writing until you truly feel finished. The lines are here to guide you, but if you feel the need to keep writing, fill in the margins. Write until you are spent. Recalling your dreams and writing about them (especially immediately after waking up) may unlock what you're truly looking for in life. When we let ourselves tap into our unconscious mind, it'll often tell us things that we avoided thinking about directly.

Symbols

HOME: Symbolizes you and how you view yourself. For example, if the house is run down, perhaps you are feeling like you're not taking care of yourself. If the house has many floors, you might feel that there are many levels to your personality and that reaching your truest self requires some climbing. The front of the house is significant to how you present yourself.

TEETH: Dreams where your teeth are falling out may mean that you are feeling powerless or are feeling a lack of stability in an area of your life. Often if you are having this dream, you are at a turning point in your life or are in the middle of a big transition.

DECEASED LOVED ONES: Depending on factors in your day-to-day life, this could mean a few different things. If the loved one or relative recently passed, this is part of the grieving process. If the person is alive in real life, you're likely considering or in the process of doing an activity that your unconscious mind associates with that person.

WATER: Corresponds to your state of mind and overall emotional well-being. Are your thoughts as tumultuous as the waves? Is the water (and your thoughts) particularly dirty? Finding that you're able to breathe underwater symbolizes power and your own ability to weather whatever it is you're currently dealing with.

NEW ROOMS: This is a wish-fulfillment dream, or a dream that gives you all that you desire. If it is a new room in your house, it could mean that there is some new part of yourself that you're very keen on having.

FOOD: Symbolizes the experiences and the energy that you're taking in. Good food means your mind is feeling nourished, while cheap food means that your mind is wanting or that a certain activity is missing from your life.

FIRE: Something in your life has become all-consuming and hungry for more. Tempers are often described as fiery, so if you find that you've been prone to anger lately, the fire in your dreams could be calling back to that.

SPIDERS: A common fear for many humans, spiders in your dreams could be linked to more irrational fears and insecurities that have been hindering your growth. Often pictured in a web, a spider can also symbolize feeling stuck or stagnant. If the spider elicits positive feelings, it could conversely revolve around something in your life that requires a lot of attention to detail and patience.

UFOS AND ALIENS: Because so little is known about both, there are many different interpretations. They could symbolize feeling untethered to the earth and a little spacey, or that you would like some sort of escape from the life you're currently living. It could also be linked to a hidden part of yourself that you're in the process of discovering. If the aliens are invading, this could be linked to your privacy being violated.

TORNADOS: If you are in a tornado during your dream, you may be feeling out of control and overwhelmed. If it's in the background of your dream, it could be related to a trend of emotional upheaval and angry outbursts.

PREGNANCY: For the most part, dreams about being pregnant are a sign that something in your life is growing and changing. There are new things coming your way. Baby dreams are typically positive and tend to symbolize new beginnings.

Themes

DRIVING: Symbolizes decision making, and the type of car can represent the type of decisions you're making. If you're dreaming that you're in a car but someone else is driving it, it means that you don't feel in control of your life. If the car you're driving is expensive or powerful, this correlates to important decisions you've made or are heading toward.

FALLING: There is a common misconception that if you hit the ground in your dream, you will die in real life, but that is not true. It can just mean that whatever is happening is out of your hands. Generally, falling dreams indicate a lack of confidence or a lack of control in your life. You may be feeling overwhelmed or struggling to break negative habits.

FLYING: Although this dream can be a little scary at first, a flying dream is usually about exploring the many freedoms and possibilities in your life. Generally, this is a positive dream that means you are in control of your life.

INTIMACY: Sex traditionally means that there's something deeply pleasurable about the goings on in your day-to-day life.

A CHASE: Being chased in a dream means that you are running from something in your life or that there might be something in your life that you are afraid to face. Knowing who is chasing you may give you a clue as to who or what you fear.

BEING TRAPPED OR LOST: These dreams can mean that you are not in control or that you may feel like you have no clear direction in an area of your life. Dreams about being trapped usually mean that you are having difficulty breaking a habit or addiction, or that someone else is in control. Dreams about being lost can mean that you are struggling to find your way through a situation.

FAILING A TEST: This a very common dream that may signify your fear of failure. It can mean you're feeling unbalanced and may need to work on getting your life back on track, or that you are lacking confidence. If you actually have a test coming up, it could be a clue from your subconscious that you forgot to study something.

LATENESS: If you dream about missing your bus, train, or airplane, you may be feeling unhappy or anxious about disappointing yourself and others in your life. It can also mean that you may need to work on your time management skills in your conscious life.

PARALYSIS: This is about feeling disenfranchised from your choices. Feeling powerless or helpless could be linked to more stimuli entering your waking life than your unconscious mind can fully process.

SEARCHING: This dream can mean that you are feeling lost or that you are missing someone in your life. Often it means that you're feeling unfulfilled in some area of your life, whether that's financial security, something within yourself, or a relationship.

NUDITY: To dream of being nude in front of people reflects your vulnerability and anxiety about how others see you. You may be hiding something that you are afraid people will be able to find out. Alternatively, if you're not hiding in shame, then it's reflecting feelings of self-confidence and self-assurance.

DEATH: While dreaming about death can be scary, this type of dream usually means the symbolic end of something and the beginning of something new. For the most part, dreaming of your death signals the resolution of a burden or the lifting of negative feelings that permits you to move forward.

MIRROR VERSIONS OF YOURSELF: It's you! Or a version of you. Mirrors often symbolize how self-aware and introspective we've become. How you interact with the mirror, or how your mirror-self acts, is correlated to how you feel about yourself and your self-confidence.

SCHOOL: Your mood while dreaming about being in school is releated to how you feel about your social life and the interactions you have with others. Is the school your elementary school? It could mean that your relationships have a carefree nature or that you're feeling like your relationships lack the maturity you're craving.

Things That Go Bump in the Night

Night terrors, anxiety dreams, and recurring dreams can all feel like fitful reasons not to sleep. They're uncomfortable and often leave you feeling more exhausted than you were when you lay down. Seeing as forgoing sleep entirely is not an option, the only way you'll ever truly learn how to overcome these pervasive feelings is to process their source. One simple way to process these themes is through this journal and by recording your dreams. Often, when we look our nightmares in the face instead of shying away from them, they don't appear as terrifying as we previously thought.

If your nightmares are particularly terrible, priming your unconscious mind with better vibes, calming imagery, and positive feelings is a good way to make the night terrors less intense. Visualization techniques can help fertilize more positive thoughts in your subconscious and can help you work through the trauma that spawns these nightmares. Use your imagination to paint calming and peaceful pictures for yourself before bed. Think about kittens, the best day you had last month, your favorite meal, and other idyllic things. It can be difficult to be positive when facing down something as unpleasant as nightmares, so start slow, have patience, and be kind to yourself.

Once you're awake, if the dregs of the nightmare are clinging to your mind, unwind them. Think about what you're grateful for to try to combat every fear that your brain generates. If your nightmares are recurring and persistent, once you've woken up and recorded them, try to reimagine more peaceful endings to traumatic dream experiences. For example, if you often dream of falling, try to restructure the dream once you're awake so that you're flying instead.

If these dreams persist even after positive visualizations, see if you can identify the source and mood while you're dreaming and ask yourself if the specific feeling or anxiety resonates with something you're familiar with in the waking world.

If nothing is working, seek the help of a professional to help guide you through the underlying trauma.

RECURRING DREAMS

If you find yourself experiencing a recurring dream, there is likely something in your life that you're not acknowledging. And by not acknowledging something your subconscious finds so obvious, you're giving yourself a bit of stress. By putting this type of coded message in your dreams, your subconscious is trying to force you to see something you're avoiding. Alternatively, there could be some past underlying trauma that your mind is still working on processing. In this case, recurring dreams tend to lessen over time.

Take both possibilities into account when trying to interpret the source of your recurring dream. If the dreams are persistent, investigate your environment to see if there are certain factors in your surroundings that could be prompting the dreams.

Although recurring dreams may have negative themes and cause the dreamer to experience stress, they're not always correlated with bad outcomes. For example, if you frequently have dreams of failing a test, you may actually do better on real examinations. These dreams are part of your brain's way of processing emotions. If you've studied hard and are deeply concerned about passing exams, this may be a habitual theme in your subconscious.

ANXIETY DREAMS / NIGHTMARES

Dreams of this variety can come in many different forms, often related to travel, work, moving, or school, among many other themes. When we feel powerless or full of anxiety in our waking life, it can often transfer into our dreams.

Anxiety dreams and nightmares may feel fairly similar to the regular dreamer. They're really only distinguishable to sleep scientists, who can chart during which piece of your sleep cycle these dreams occur. Incomplete tasks and a sense of helplessness are common themes in anxiety dreams.

Our dreams are where our subconscious mind picks apart the different things that bothered us during the day, deep down. In this light, having anxious dreams isn't uncommon. There will always be something to trouble you, but it's important to remember that these anxiety dreams often serve a purpose. Being anxious about travel will likely make you more alert and less likely to forget crucial items for your trip when you're leaving the house. Work stress dreams may be your mind trying to work out the things that stress you out or slow you down while you're asleep so that work can be less stressful overall.

Anxiety dreams are normal and it's important not to let them cause you extra worry.

Night Terrors

Night terrors are aptly named and bring about intense or agonizing dread in the dreamer. The traditional difference between anxiety dreams and night terrors is that night terrors will wake you up from a dead sleep. Night terrors occur before you reach REM, and so will hinder you from good sleep. They can be paired with sleep walking, thrashing, and partial arousal from sleep. These episodes typically only last between 5 and 30 minutes, with the sleeper (hopefully) finding their way back to bed and sleep.

Most commonly occurring in children, night terrors can be caused by fever, stress, sleep deprivation, depression, anxiety, or alcohol use, and can also be the side effect of some medications.

Night terrors can also be the result of eating later in the evening. The digestion process signals the brain to be more active, and when the rest of the body is dormant this activity can be set loose in your nightmares.

These dreams can include physical sensations like a weight on your chest or shortness of breath. If you do feel a weight on your chest while you're dreaming or have difficulty breathing while you're sleeping, you should consult your physician. Night terrors will usually subside over time, but if they persist, it's best to talk to a doctor.

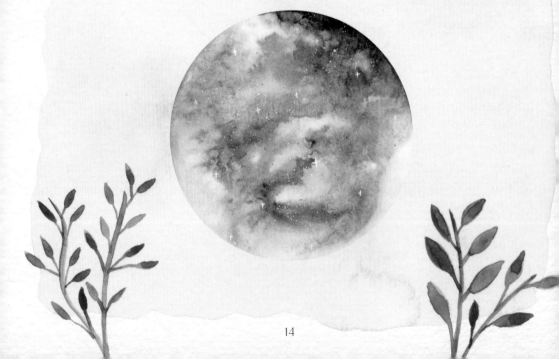

Recalling Your Dreams

Dreams are often gifts of insight from our subconscious, but they can be elusive and difficult to pin down. Here are a few tips on how to draw them out.

PREPARE TO RECORD your dream. Keep a pen and this journal right by your bedside. An hour before bed, plug your phone in and don't look at it again until after you've recorded your dreams. Disconnecting from your screens and the blue light that they emit will cue your brain into the fact that it's time to sleep. Do your best to get 7–8 hours of sleep a night. Giving yourself enough time to venture into the REM phase of sleep will make you feel more rested the next day, and easing yourself out of your dreams will be less jarring.

DIRECTLY BEFORE BED remind your subconscious that you want to record your dream in the morning. Tell yourself that you're going to remember your dreams. Repeat this a few times to solidify your intention while you drift off. Take some time to relax your mind and bring your consciousness into a peaceful place. If you're prone to nightmares, try visualizing peaceful scenes that make your muscles relax. Happy memories, pleasant vistas, soothing water sounds…anything that'll bring a sense of harmony to your busy mind.

IMMEDIATELY AFTER WAKING, when the dregs of the dream are still clinging to your mind, record your dream. Try not to activate your mind. Staying in this limbo between the waking world and dreamland will make it easier for you to remember the details of your dreams.

BE PATIENT with yourself as you begin this journey. Don't force your memory. The more you force your conscious mind on your dreams, the more elusive they become. If all that comes to you are snippets and images, take those gifts and work with them. The more you practice recording your dreams, the easier and more fluid the experience will become.

REPEAT, REPEAT, REPEAT. Form a habit of recording your dreams for the best results. The more frequently you analyze your dreams, the easier it will become. If your unconscious mind grows used to recording your dreams on a nightly basis, recalling your dreams will become second nature.

INTERPRETING YOUR DREAMS

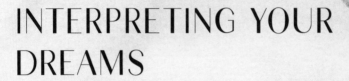

Break down your dreams into manageable parts. Pull them apart, piece by piece, to make sure that you don't miss anything.

Is there a narrative? What order did they come in? Were there many different settings? Do you categorize each new location and cast of characters as a different dream? What mood were you in while you were dreaming? Were there any intense physical sensations?

Make note of how the different parts interact with one another. The language of your dreams is often hidden in the subtle ways that the pieces fit together.

What moods corresponded to each setting? Did any of the characters change their face but elicit the same feelings of attachment?

Look for common themes. If a certain character, location, or theme keeps popping up, there's something in your waking life that is likely plaguing your subconscious.

Is the same person visiting you in your dreams from night to night? Do the same landmarks keep reappearing on your journey? Are people repeating the same phrase or word, even when it seems out of place?

Colors and numbers have their own significance, so if any jump out at you, document them in detail.

All the information provided here is only a lightning rod. If the interpretations offered in the book don't resonate, perhaps your subconscious is being more literal. More important than the symbology of the imagery is how the dream made you feel.

Sample Dream

You're in college and are on your way to class. As you cross the great lawn, all of the pathways are now made of water and you're feeling a little panicked as your normal walk to class is now difficult terrain.

School symbolizes a social interaction. University typically symbolizes a more carefree time.

The pathways symbolize the way you're supposed to be going.

Having the pathways transform into water means that you're feeling emotional about the route that you're supposed to be taking.

By tying these three themes together, you can link your dreams to a situation you're currently experiencing. Perhaps you are emotional about not being as carefree in your social life as you were previously and it is leaving you feeling confused about how to proceed.

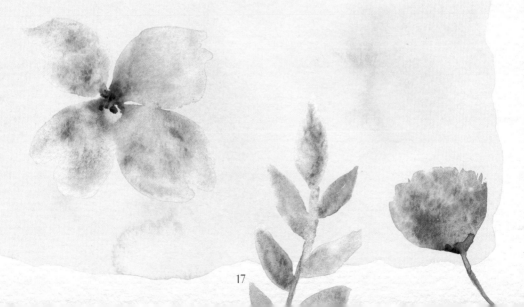

Dream

Date: ....

TYPE OF DREAM

★ First-time Dream   ★ Recurring Dream

★ Scary Dream   ★ Adventurous Dream

★ Happy Dream   ★ Unique Dream

THEMES

★ Driving   ★ Lateness

★ Falling   ★ Paralysis

★ Flying   ★ Searching

★ Intimacy   ★ Nudity

★ A Chase   ★ Death

★ Trapped / Lost   ★ Mirror

★ Failing   ★ School

How did this dream make you feel when you woke up?

_____

_____

_____

Description of the dream.

_____

_____

_____

_____

_____

If this is a recurring dream, was there anything different that you can remember happened this time? If not, what common things do you always see in the dream?

_____

_____

_____

_____

What types of sights, scents, or sounds do you remember most from the dream?

_____

_____

_____

_____

What three things do you remember the most from the dream?

_____

_____

_____

_____

How would you interpret this dream in relation to your life and personality?

_____

_____

_____

_____

What was the overall emotion in the dream?

_____

_____

_____

_____

What do you think is the overall message?

_____

_____

_____

What actions will you take in your daily life?

_____

_____

_____

_____

_____

_____

Draw the most memorable scene or symbol from your dream.

Dream

Date: ....

TYPE OF DREAM

⭐ First-time Dream

⭐ Scary Dream

⭐ Happy Dream

⭐ Recurring Dream

⭐ Adventurous Dream

⭐ Unique Dream

THEMES

⭐ Driving

⭐ Falling

⭐ Flying

⭐ Intimacy

⭐ A Chase

⭐ Trapped / Lost

⭐ Failing

⭐ Lateness

⭐ Paralysis

⭐ Searching

⭐ Nudity

⭐ Death

⭐ Mirror

⭐ School

How did this dream make you feel when you woke up?

_____

_____

_____

Description of the dream.

_____

_____

_____

_____

_____

If this is a recurring dream, was there anything different that you can remember happened this time? If not, what common things do you always see in the dream?

_____

_____

_____

_____

_____

What types of sights, scents, or sounds do you remember most from the dream?

_____

_____

_____

_____

_____

What three things do you remember the most from the dream?

_____

_____

_____

_____

How would you interpret this dream in relation to your life and personality?

_____

_____

_____

_____

What was the overall emotion in the dream?

_____

_____

_____

_____

What do you think is the overall message?

_____

_____

_____

What actions will you take in your daily life?

_____

_____

_____

_____

_____

Draw the most memorable scene or symbol from your dream.

Dream

Date: ....

TYPE OF DREAM

★ First-time Dream

★ Scary Dream

★ Happy Dream

★ Recurring Dream

★ Adventurous Dream

★ Unique Dream

THEMES

★ Driving

★ Falling

★ Flying

★ Intimacy

★ A Chase

★ Trapped / Lost

★ Failing

★ Lateness

★ Paralysis

★ Searching

★ Nudity

★ Death

★ Mirror

★ School

How did this dream make you feel when you woke up?

_____

_____

_____

Description of the dream.

_____

_____

_____

_____

_____

If this is a recurring dream, was there anything different that you can remember happened this time? If not, what common things do you always see in the dream?

_____

_____

_____

_____

_____

What types of sights, scents, or sounds do you remember most from the dream?

_____

_____

_____

_____

_____

What three things do you remember the most from the dream?

How would you interpret this dream in relation to your life and personality?

What was the overall emotion in the dream?

What do you think is the overall message?

What actions will you take in your daily life?

_____

_____

_____

_____

_____

_____

Draw the most memorable scene or symbol from your dream.

Dream

Date: ....

TYPE OF DREAM

★ First-time Dream   ★ Recurring Dream

★ Scary Dream   ★ Adventurous Dream

★ Happy Dream   ★ Unique Dream

THEMES

★ Driving   ★ Lateness

★ Falling   ★ Paralysis

★ Flying   ★ Searching

★ Intimacy   ★ Nudity

★ A Chase   ★ Death

★ Trapped / Lost   ★ Mirror

★ Failing   ★ School

How did this dream make you feel when you woke up?

_____

_____

_____

Description of the dream.

_____

_____

_____

_____

_____

If this is a recurring dream, was there anything different that you can remember happened this time? If not, what common things do you always see in the dream?

_____

_____

_____

_____

_____

What types of sights, scents, or sounds do you remember most from the dream?

_____

_____

_____

_____

_____

What three things do you remember the most from the dream?

_____

_____

_____

_____

How would you interpret this dream in relation to your life and personality?

_____

_____

_____

_____

What was the overall emotion in the dream?

_____

_____

_____

_____

What do you think is the overall message?

_____

_____

_____

What actions will you take in your daily life?

_____

_____

_____

_____

_____

_____

Draw the most memorable scene or symbol from your dream.

Dream

Date: ....

TYPE OF DREAM

⭐ First-time Dream   ⭐ Recurring Dream

⭐ Scary Dream   ⭐ Adventurous Dream

⭐ Happy Dream   ⭐ Unique Dream

THEMES

⭐ Driving   ⭐ Lateness

⭐ Falling   ⭐ Paralysis

⭐ Flying   ⭐ Searching

⭐ Intimacy   ⭐ Nudity

⭐ A Chase   ⭐ Death

⭐ Trapped / Lost   ⭐ Mirror

⭐ Failing   ⭐ School

How did this dream make you feel when you woke up?

_____

_____

_____

Description of the dream.

_____

_____

_____

_____

_____

If this is a recurring dream, was there anything different that you can remember happened this time? If not, what common things do you always see in the dream?

_____

_____

_____

_____

What types of sights, scents, or sounds do you remember most from the dream?

_____

_____

_____

_____

What three things do you remember the most from the dream?

_____

_____

_____

_____

How would you interpret this dream in relation to your life and personality?

_____

_____

_____

_____

What was the overall emotion in the dream?

_____

_____

_____

_____

What do you think is the overall message?

_____

_____

_____

What actions will you take in your daily life?

_____

_____

_____

_____

_____

Draw the most memorable scene or symbol from your dream.

Dream

Date: ....

TYPE OF DREAM

⭐ First-time Dream

⭐ Scary Dream

⭐ Happy Dream

⭐ Recurring Dream

⭐ Adventurous Dream

⭐ Unique Dream

THEMES

⭐ Driving

⭐ Falling

⭐ Flying

⭐ Intimacy

⭐ A Chase

⭐ Trapped / Lost

⭐ Failing

⭐ Lateness

⭐ Paralysis

⭐ Searching

⭐ Nudity

⭐ Death

⭐ Mirror

⭐ School

How did this dream make you feel when you woke up?

_____

_____

_____

Description of the dream.

_____

_____

_____

_____

If this is a recurring dream, was there anything different that you can remember happened this time? If not, what common things do you always see in the dream?

_____

_____

_____

_____

What types of sights, scents, or sounds do you remember most from the dream?

_____

_____

_____

_____

What three things do you remember the most from the dream?

_____

_____

_____

_____

How would you interpret this dream in relation to your life and personality?

_____

_____

_____

_____

What was the overall emotion in the dream?

_____

_____

_____

_____

What do you think is the overall message?

_____

_____

_____

What actions will you take in your daily life?

_____

_____

_____

_____

_____

_____

Draw the most memorable scene or symbol from your dream.

Dream

Date: ....

TYPE OF DREAM

⭐ First-time Dream

⭐ Scary Dream

⭐ Happy Dream

⭐ Recurring Dream

⭐ Adventurous Dream

⭐ Unique Dream

THEMES

⭐ Driving

⭐ Falling

⭐ Flying

⭐ Intimacy

⭐ A Chase

⭐ Trapped / Lost

⭐ Failing

⭐ Lateness

⭐ Paralysis

⭐ Searching

⭐ Nudity

⭐ Death

⭐ Mirror

⭐ School

How did this dream make you feel when you woke up?

_____

_____

_____

Description of the dream.

_____

_____

_____

_____

_____

If this is a recurring dream, was there anything different that you can remember happened this time? If not, what common things do you always see in the dream?

_____

_____

_____

_____

_____

What types of sights, scents, or sounds do you remember most from the dream?

_____

_____

_____

_____

What three things do you remember the most from the dream?

_____

_____

_____

_____

How would you interpret this dream in relation to your life and personality?

_____

_____

_____

_____

What was the overall emotion in the dream?

_____

_____

_____

_____

What do you think is the overall message?

_____

_____

_____

What actions will you take in your daily life?

_____

_____

_____

_____

_____

Draw the most memorable scene or symbol from your dream.

Dream

Date: ....

TYPE OF DREAM

★ First-time Dream

★ Scary Dream

★ Happy Dream

★ Recurring Dream

★ Adventurous Dream

★ Unique Dream

THEMES

★ Driving

★ Falling

★ Flying

★ Intimacy

★ A Chase

★ Trapped / Lost

★ Failing

★ Lateness

★ Paralysis

★ Searching

★ Nudity

★ Death

★ Mirror

★ School

How did this dream make you feel when you woke up?

_____

_____

_____

Description of the dream.

_____

_____

_____

_____

_____

If this is a recurring dream, was there anything different that you can remember happened this time? If not, what common things do you always see in the dream?

_____

_____

_____

_____

What types of sights, scents, or sounds do you remember most from the dream?

_____

_____

_____

_____

What three things do you remember the most from the dream?

_____

_____

_____

_____

How would you interpret this dream in relation to your life and personality?

_____

_____

_____

_____

What was the overall emotion in the dream?

_____

_____

_____

_____

What do you think is the overall message?

_____

_____

_____

What actions will you take in your daily life?

_____

_____

_____

_____

_____

_____

Draw the most memorable scene or symbol from your dream.

Dream

Date: ....

TYPE OF DREAM

- ⭐ First-time Dream
- ⭐ Scary Dream
- ⭐ Happy Dream

- ⭐ Recurring Dream
- ⭐ Adventurous Dream
- ⭐ Unique Dream

THEMES

- ⭐ Driving
- ⭐ Falling
- ⭐ Flying
- ⭐ Intimacy
- ⭐ A Chase
- ⭐ Trapped / Lost
- ⭐ Failing

- ⭐ Lateness
- ⭐ Paralysis
- ⭐ Searching
- ⭐ Nudity
- ⭐ Death
- ⭐ Mirror
- ⭐ School

How did this dream make you feel when you woke up?

_____

_____

_____

Description of the dream.

_____

_____

_____

_____

If this is a recurring dream, was there anything different that you can remember happened this time? If not, what common things do you always see in the dream?

_____

_____

_____

_____

What types of sights, scents, or sounds do you remember most from the dream?

_____

_____

_____

_____

What three things do you remember the most from the dream?

_____

_____

_____

_____

How would you interpret this dream in relation to your life and personality?

_____

_____

_____

_____

What was the overall emotion in the dream?

_____

_____

_____

_____

What do you think is the overall message?

_____

_____

_____

What actions will you take in your daily life?

_____

_____

_____

_____

_____

_____

Draw the most memorable scene or symbol from your dream.

Dream

Date: ....

TYPE OF DREAM

⭐ First-time Dream   ⭐ Recurring Dream

⭐ Scary Dream   ⭐ Adventurous Dream

⭐ Happy Dream   ⭐ Unique Dream

THEMES

⭐ Driving   ⭐ Lateness

⭐ Falling   ⭐ Paralysis

⭐ Flying   ⭐ Searching

⭐ Intimacy   ⭐ Nudity

⭐ A Chase   ⭐ Death

⭐ Trapped / Lost   ⭐ Mirror

⭐ Failing   ⭐ School

How did this dream make you feel when you woke up?

_____

_____

_____

Description of the dream.

_____

_____

_____

_____

_____

If this is a recurring dream, was there anything different that you can remember happened this time? If not, what common things do you always see in the dream?

_____

_____

_____

_____

_____

What types of sights, scents, or sounds do you remember most from the dream?

_____

_____

_____

_____

_____

What three things do you remember the most from the dream?

_____

_____

_____

_____

How would you interpret this dream in relation to your life and personality?

_____

_____

_____

_____

What was the overall emotion in the dream?

_____

_____

_____

_____

What do you think is the overall message?

_____

_____

_____

What actions will you take in your daily life?

_____

_____

_____

_____

_____

Draw the most memorable scene or symbol from your dream.

Dream

Date: ....

TYPE OF DREAM

★ First-time Dream

★ Scary Dream

★ Happy Dream

★ Recurring Dream

★ Adventurous Dream

★ Unique Dream

THEMES

★ Driving

★ Falling

★ Flying

★ Intimacy

★ A Chase

★ Trapped / Lost

★ Failing

★ Lateness

★ Paralysis

★ Searching

★ Nudity

★ Death

★ Mirror

★ School

How did this dream make you feel when you woke up?

_____

_____

_____

Description of the dream.

_____

_____

_____

_____

_____

If this is a recurring dream, was there anything different that you can remember happened this time? If not, what common things do you always see in the dream?

_____

_____

_____

_____

_____

What types of sights, scents, or sounds do you remember most from the dream?

_____

_____

_____

_____

What three things do you remember the most from the dream?

_____

_____

_____

_____

How would you interpret this dream in relation to your life and personality?

_____

_____

_____

_____

What was the overall emotion in the dream?

_____

_____

_____

_____

What do you think is the overall message?

_____

_____

_____

What actions will you take in your daily life?

_____

_____

_____

_____

_____

Draw the most memorable scene or symbol from your dream.

Dream

Date: ....

TYPE OF DREAM

⭐ First-time Dream   ⭐ Recurring Dream

⭐ Scary Dream   ⭐ Adventurous Dream

⭐ Happy Dream   ⭐ Unique Dream

THEMES

⭐ Driving   ⭐ Lateness

⭐ Falling   ⭐ Paralysis

⭐ Flying   ⭐ Searching

⭐ Intimacy   ⭐ Nudity

⭐ A Chase   ⭐ Death

⭐ Trapped / Lost   ⭐ Mirror

⭐ Failing   ⭐ School

How did this dream make you feel when you woke up?

_____

_____

_____

Description of the dream.

_____

_____

_____

_____

_____

If this is a recurring dream, was there anything different that you can remember happened this time? If not, what common things do you always see in the dream?

_____

_____

_____

_____

What types of sights, scents, or sounds do you remember most from the dream?

_____

_____

_____

_____

What three things do you remember the most from the dream?

_____

_____

_____

_____

How would you interpret this dream in relation to your life and personality?

_____

_____

_____

_____

What was the overall emotion in the dream?

_____

_____

_____

_____

What do you think is the overall message?

_____

_____

_____

What actions will you take in your daily life?

_____

_____

_____

_____

_____

Draw the most memorable scene or symbol from your dream.

Dream

Date: ....

TYPE OF DREAM

⭐ First-time Dream   ⭐ Recurring Dream

⭐ Scary Dream   ⭐ Adventurous Dream

⭐ Happy Dream   ⭐ Unique Dream

THEMES

⭐ Driving   ⭐ Lateness

⭐ Falling   ⭐ Paralysis

⭐ Flying   ⭐ Searching

⭐ Intimacy   ⭐ Nudity

⭐ A Chase   ⭐ Death

⭐ Trapped / Lost   ⭐ Mirror

⭐ Failing   ⭐ School

How did this dream make you feel when you woke up?

_____

_____

_____

Description of the dream.

_____

_____

_____

_____

_____

If this is a recurring dream, was there anything different that you can remember happened this time? If not, what common things do you always see in the dream?

_____

_____

_____

_____

What types of sights, scents, or sounds do you remember most from the dream?

_____

_____

_____

_____

What three things do you remember the most from the dream?

_____

_____

_____

_____

How would you interpret this dream in relation to your life and personality?

_____

_____

_____

_____

What was the overall emotion in the dream?

_____

_____

_____

_____

What do you think is the overall message?

_____

_____

_____

What actions will you take in your daily life?

_____

_____

_____

_____

_____

_____

Draw the most memorable scene or symbol from your dream.

Dream

Date: ....

TYPE OF DREAM

★ First-time Dream   ★ Recurring Dream

★ Scary Dream   ★ Adventurous Dream

★ Happy Dream   ★ Unique Dream

THEMES

★ Driving   ★ Lateness

★ Falling   ★ Paralysis

★ Flying   ★ Searching

★ Intimacy   ★ Nudity

★ A Chase   ★ Death

★ Trapped / Lost   ★ Mirror

★ Failing   ★ School

How did this dream make you feel when you woke up?

_____

_____

_____

Description of the dream.

_____

_____

_____

_____

If this is a recurring dream, was there anything different that you can remember happened this time? If not, what common things do you always see in the dream?

_____

_____

_____

_____

What types of sights, scents, or sounds do you remember most from the dream?

_____

_____

_____

_____

What three things do you remember the most from the dream?

_____

_____

_____

_____

How would you interpret this dream in relation to your life and personality?

_____

_____

_____

_____

What was the overall emotion in the dream?

_____

_____

_____

_____

What do you think is the overall message?

_____

_____

_____

_____

What actions will you take in your daily life?

_____

_____

_____

_____

_____

Draw the most memorable scene or symbol from your dream.

Dream

Date: ....

TYPE OF DREAM

⭐ First-time Dream   ⭐ Recurring Dream

⭐ Scary Dream   ⭐ Adventurous Dream

⭐ Happy Dream   ⭐ Unique Dream

THEMES

⭐ Driving   ⭐ Lateness

⭐ Falling   ⭐ Paralysis

⭐ Flying   ⭐ Searching

⭐ Intimacy   ⭐ Nudity

⭐ A Chase   ⭐ Death

⭐ Trapped / Lost   ⭐ Mirror

⭐ Failing   ⭐ School

How did this dream make you feel when you woke up?

....

....

....

Description of the dream.

_____

_____

_____

_____

If this is a recurring dream, was there anything different that you can remember happened this time? If not, what common things do you always see in the dream?

_____

_____

_____

_____

What types of sights, scents, or sounds do you remember most from the dream?

_____

_____

_____

_____

What three things do you remember the most from the dream?

_____

_____

_____

_____

How would you interpret this dream in relation to your life and personality?

_____

_____

_____

_____

What was the overall emotion in the dream?

_____

_____

_____

_____

What do you think is the overall message?

_____

_____

_____

_____

What actions will you take in your daily life?

_____

_____

_____

_____

_____

_____

Draw the most memorable scene or symbol from your dream.

Dream

Date: ....

TYPE OF DREAM

⭐ First-time Dream

⭐ Scary Dream

⭐ Happy Dream

⭐ Recurring Dream

⭐ Adventurous Dream

⭐ Unique Dream

THEMES

⭐ Driving

⭐ Falling

⭐ Flying

⭐ Intimacy

⭐ A Chase

⭐ Trapped / Lost

⭐ Failing

⭐ Lateness

⭐ Paralysis

⭐ Searching

⭐ Nudity

⭐ Death

⭐ Mirror

⭐ School

How did this dream make you feel when you woke up?

_____

_____

_____

Description of the dream.

_____

_____

_____

_____

_____

If this is a recurring dream, was there anything different that you can remember happened this time? If not, what common things do you always see in the dream?

_____

_____

_____

_____

What types of sights, scents, or sounds do you remember most from the dream?

_____

_____

_____

_____

What three things do you remember the most from the dream?

_____

_____

_____

_____

How would you interpret this dream in relation to your life and personality?

_____

_____

_____

_____

What was the overall emotion in the dream?

_____

_____

_____

_____

What do you think is the overall message?

_____

_____

_____

What actions will you take in your daily life?

_____

_____

_____

_____

_____

Draw the most memorable scene or symbol from your dream.

Dream

Date: ....

TYPE OF DREAM

⭐ First-time Dream   ⭐ Recurring Dream

⭐ Scary Dream   ⭐ Adventurous Dream

⭐ Happy Dream   ⭐ Unique Dream

THEMES

⭐ Driving   ⭐ Lateness

⭐ Falling   ⭐ Paralysis

⭐ Flying   ⭐ Searching

⭐ Intimacy   ⭐ Nudity

⭐ A Chase   ⭐ Death

⭐ Trapped / Lost   ⭐ Mirror

⭐ Failing   ⭐ School

How did this dream make you feel when you woke up?

_____

_____

_____

Description of the dream.

_____

_____

_____

_____

If this is a recurring dream, was there anything different that you can remember happened this time? If not, what common things do you always see in the dream?

_____

_____

_____

_____

What types of sights, scents, or sounds do you remember most from the dream?

_____

_____

_____

_____

What three things do you remember the most from the dream?

_____

_____

_____

_____

How would you interpret this dream in relation to your life and personality?

_____

_____

_____

_____

What was the overall emotion in the dream?

_____

_____

_____

_____

What do you think is the overall message?

_____

_____

_____

What actions will you take in your daily life?

_____

_____

_____

_____

_____

_____

Draw the most memorable scene or symbol from your dream.

Dream

Date: ....

TYPE OF DREAM

★ First-time Dream   ★ Recurring Dream

★ Scary Dream   ★ Adventurous Dream

★ Happy Dream   ★ Unique Dream

THEMES

★ Driving   ★ Lateness

★ Falling   ★ Paralysis

★ Flying   ★ Searching

★ Intimacy   ★ Nudity

★ A Chase   ★ Death

★ Trapped / Lost   ★ Mirror

★ Failing   ★ School

How did this dream make you feel when you woke up?

_____

_____

_____

Description of the dream.

_____

_____

_____

_____

_____

If this is a recurring dream, was there anything different that you can remember happened this time? If not, what common things do you always see in the dream?

_____

_____

_____

_____

What types of sights, scents, or sounds do you remember most from the dream?

_____

_____

_____

_____

What three things do you remember the most from the dream?

_____

_____

_____

_____

How would you interpret this dream in relation to your life and personality?

_____

_____

_____

_____

What was the overall emotion in the dream?

_____

_____

_____

_____

What do you think is the overall message?

_____

_____

_____

What actions will you take in your daily life?

_____

_____

_____

_____

_____

_____

Draw the most memorable scene or symbol from your dream.

Dream

Date: ....

TYPE OF DREAM

★ First-time Dream

★ Scary Dream

★ Happy Dream

★ Recurring Dream

★ Adventurous Dream

★ Unique Dream

THEMES

★ Driving

★ Falling

★ Flying

★ Intimacy

★ A Chase

★ Trapped / Lost

★ Failing

★ Lateness

★ Paralysis

★ Searching

★ Nudity

★ Death

★ Mirror

★ School

How did this dream make you feel when you woke up?

_____

_____

_____

Description of the dream.

_____

_____

_____

_____

_____

If this is a recurring dream, was there anything different that you can remember happened this time? If not, what common things do you always see in the dream?

_____

_____

_____

_____

What types of sights, scents, or sounds do you remember most from the dream?

_____

_____

_____

_____

What three things do you remember the most from the dream?

_____

_____

_____

_____

How would you interpret this dream in relation to your life and personality?

_____

_____

_____

_____

What was the overall emotion in the dream?

_____

_____

_____

_____

What do you think is the overall message?

_____

_____

_____

What actions will you take in your daily life?

_____

_____

_____

_____

_____

Draw the most memorable scene or symbol from your dream.

Dream

Date: ....

TYPE OF DREAM

★ First-time Dream

★ Scary Dream

★ Happy Dream

★ Recurring Dream

★ Adventurous Dream

★ Unique Dream

THEMES

★ Driving

★ Falling

★ Flying

★ Intimacy

★ A Chase

★ Trapped / Lost

★ Failing

★ Lateness

★ Paralysis

★ Searching

★ Nudity

★ Death

★ Mirror

★ School

How did this dream make you feel when you woke up?

_____

_____

_____

Description of the dream.

_____

_____

_____

_____

If this is a recurring dream, was there anything different that you can remember happened this time? If not, what common things do you always see in the dream?

_____

_____

_____

_____

What types of sights, scents, or sounds do you remember most from the dream?

_____

_____

_____

_____

What three things do you remember the most from the dream?

_____

_____

_____

_____

How would you interpret this dream in relation to your life and personality?

_____

_____

_____

_____

What was the overall emotion in the dream?

_____

_____

_____

_____

What do you think is the overall message?

_____

_____

_____

_____

What actions will you take in your daily life?

_____

_____

_____

_____

_____

Draw the most memorable scene or symbol from your dream.

Dream

Date: ....

TYPE OF DREAM

⭐ First-time Dream   ⭐ Recurring Dream

⭐ Scary Dream   ⭐ Adventurous Dream

⭐ Happy Dream   ⭐ Unique Dream

THEMES

⭐ Driving   ⭐ Lateness

⭐ Falling   ⭐ Paralysis

⭐ Flying   ⭐ Searching

⭐ Intimacy   ⭐ Nudity

⭐ A Chase   ⭐ Death

⭐ Trapped / Lost   ⭐ Mirror

⭐ Failing   ⭐ School

How did this dream make you feel when you woke up?

_____

_____

_____

Description of the dream.

_____

_____

_____

_____

_____

If this is a recurring dream, was there anything different that you can remember happened this time? If not, what common things do you always see in the dream?

_____

_____

_____

_____

What types of sights, scents, or sounds do you remember most from the dream?

_____

_____

_____

_____

What three things do you remember the most from the dream?

_____

_____

_____

_____

How would you interpret this dream in relation to your life and personality?

_____

_____

_____

_____

What was the overall emotion in the dream?

_____

_____

_____

_____

What do you think is the overall message?

_____

_____

_____

What actions will you take in your daily life?

_____

_____

_____

_____

_____

_____

Draw the most memorable scene or symbol from your dream.

Dream

Date: ....

TYPE OF DREAM

⭐ First-time Dream   ⭐ Recurring Dream

⭐ Scary Dream   ⭐ Adventurous Dream

⭐ Happy Dream   ⭐ Unique Dream

THEMES

⭐ Driving   ⭐ Lateness

⭐ Falling   ⭐ Paralysis

⭐ Flying   ⭐ Searching

⭐ Intimacy   ⭐ Nudity

⭐ A Chase   ⭐ Death

⭐ Trapped / Lost   ⭐ Mirror

⭐ Failing   ⭐ School

How did this dream make you feel when you woke up?

_____

_____

_____

Description of the dream.

_____

_____

_____

_____

If this is a recurring dream, was there anything different that you can remember happened this time? If not, what common things do you always see in the dream?

_____

_____

_____

_____

What types of sights, scents, or sounds do you remember most from the dream?

_____

_____

_____

_____

What three things do you remember the most from the dream?

_____

_____

_____

_____

How would you interpret this dream in relation to your life and personality?

_____

_____

_____

_____

What was the overall emotion in the dream?

_____

_____

_____

_____

What do you think is the overall message?

_____

_____

_____

What actions will you take in your daily life?

_____

_____

_____

_____

_____

_____

Draw the most memorable scene or symbol from your dream.

Dream

Date: ....

TYPE OF DREAM

⭐ First-time Dream

⭐ Scary Dream

⭐ Happy Dream

⭐ Recurring Dream

⭐ Adventurous Dream

⭐ Unique Dream

THEMES

⭐ Driving

⭐ Falling

⭐ Flying

⭐ Intimacy

⭐ A Chase

⭐ Trapped / Lost

⭐ Failing

⭐ Lateness

⭐ Paralysis

⭐ Searching

⭐ Nudity

⭐ Death

⭐ Mirror

⭐ School

How did this dream make you feel when you woke up?

_____

_____

_____

Description of the dream.

_____

_____

_____

_____

If this is a recurring dream, was there anything different that you can remember happened this time? If not, what common things do you always see in the dream?

_____

_____

_____

_____

What types of sights, scents, or sounds do you remember most from the dream?

_____

_____

_____

_____

What three things do you remember the most from the dream?

_____

_____

_____

_____

How would you interpret this dream in relation to your life and personality?

_____

_____

_____

_____

What was the overall emotion in the dream?

_____

_____

_____

_____

What do you think is the overall message?

_____

_____

_____

What actions will you take in your daily life?

_____

_____

_____

_____

_____

_____

Draw the most memorable scene or symbol from your dream.

Dream

Date: ....

TYPE OF DREAM

⭐ First-time Dream   ⭐ Recurring Dream

⭐ Scary Dream   ⭐ Adventurous Dream

⭐ Happy Dream   ⭐ Unique Dream

THEMES

⭐ Driving   ⭐ Lateness

⭐ Falling   ⭐ Paralysis

⭐ Flying   ⭐ Searching

⭐ Intimacy   ⭐ Nudity

⭐ A Chase   ⭐ Death

⭐ Trapped / Lost   ⭐ Mirror

⭐ Failing   ⭐ School

How did this dream make you feel when you woke up?

_____

_____

_____

Description of the dream.

_____

_____

_____

_____

If this is a recurring dream, was there anything different that you can remember happened this time? If not, what common things do you always see in the dream?

_____

_____

_____

_____

What types of sights, scents, or sounds do you remember most from the dream?

_____

_____

_____

_____

What three things do you remember the most from the dream?

_____

_____

_____

_____

How would you interpret this dream in relation to your life and personality?

_____

_____

_____

_____

What was the overall emotion in the dream?

_____

_____

_____

_____

What do you think is the overall message?

_____

_____

_____

What actions will you take in your daily life?

_____

_____

_____

_____

_____

_____

Draw the most memorable scene or symbol from your dream.

Dream

Date: ....

TYPE OF DREAM

★ First-time Dream

★ Scary Dream

★ Happy Dream

★ Recurring Dream

★ Adventurous Dream

★ Unique Dream

THEMES

★ Driving

★ Falling

★ Flying

★ Intimacy

★ A Chase

★ Trapped / Lost

★ Failing

★ Lateness

★ Paralysis

★ Searching

★ Nudity

★ Death

★ Mirror

★ School

How did this dream make you feel when you woke up?

_____

_____

_____

Description of the dream.

_____

_____

_____

_____

_____

If this is a recurring dream, was there anything different that you can remember happened this time? If not, what common things do you always see in the dream?

_____

_____

_____

_____

_____

What types of sights, scents, or sounds do you remember most from the dream?

_____

_____

_____

_____

What three things do you remember the most from the dream?

_____

_____

_____

_____

How would you interpret this dream in relation to your life and personality?

_____

_____

_____

_____

What was the overall emotion in the dream?

_____

_____

_____

_____

What do you think is the overall message?

_____

_____

_____

What actions will you take in your daily life?

_____

_____

_____

_____

_____

Draw the most memorable scene or symbol from your dream.

Dream

Date: ....

TYPE OF DREAM

⭐ First-time Dream

⭐ Scary Dream

⭐ Happy Dream

⭐ Recurring Dream

⭐ Adventurous Dream

⭐ Unique Dream

THEMES

⭐ Driving

⭐ Falling

⭐ Flying

⭐ Intimacy

⭐ A Chase

⭐ Trapped / Lost

⭐ Failing

⭐ Lateness

⭐ Paralysis

⭐ Searching

⭐ Nudity

⭐ Death

⭐ Mirror

⭐ School

How did this dream make you feel when you woke up?

_____

_____

_____

Description of the dream.

_____

_____

_____

_____

_____

If this is a recurring dream, was there anything different that you can remember happened this time? If not, what common things do you always see in the dream?

_____

_____

_____

_____

What types of sights, scents, or sounds do you remember most from the dream?

_____

_____

_____

_____

What three things do you remember the most from the dream?

_____

_____

_____

_____

How would you interpret this dream in relation to your life and personality?

_____

_____

_____

_____

What was the overall emotion in the dream?

_____

_____

_____

_____

What do you think is the overall message?

_____

_____

_____

_____

What actions will you take in your daily life?

_____

_____

_____

_____

_____

_____

_____

Draw the most memorable scene or symbol from your dream.

Dream

Date: ....

TYPE OF DREAM

★ First-time Dream

★ Scary Dream

★ Happy Dream

★ Recurring Dream

★ Adventurous Dream

★ Unique Dream

THEMES

★ Driving

★ Falling

★ Flying

★ Intimacy

★ A Chase

★ Trapped / Lost

★ Failing

★ Lateness

★ Paralysis

★ Searching

★ Nudity

★ Death

★ Mirror

★ School

How did this dream make you feel when you woke up?

_____

_____

_____

Description of the dream.

_____

_____

_____

_____

If this is a recurring dream, was there anything different that you can remember happened this time? If not, what common things do you always see in the dream?

_____

_____

_____

_____

What types of sights, scents, or sounds do you remember most from the dream?

_____

_____

_____

_____

What three things do you remember the most from the dream?

_____

_____

_____

_____

How would you interpret this dream in relation to your life and personality?

_____

_____

_____

_____

What was the overall emotion in the dream?

_____

_____

_____

_____

What do you think is the overall message?

_____

_____

_____

What actions will you take in your daily life?

_____

_____

_____

_____

_____

_____

Draw the most memorable scene or symbol from your dream.

Dream

Date: ....

TYPE OF DREAM

★ First-time Dream

★ Scary Dream

★ Happy Dream

★ Recurring Dream

★ Adventurous Dream

★ Unique Dream

THEMES

★ Driving

★ Falling

★ Flying

★ Intimacy

★ A Chase

★ Trapped / Lost

★ Failing

★ Lateness

★ Paralysis

★ Searching

★ Nudity

★ Death

★ Mirror

★ School

How did this dream make you feel when you woke up?

_____

_____

_____

Description of the dream.

_____

_____

_____

_____

If this is a recurring dream, was there anything different that you can remember happened this time? If not, what common things do you always see in the dream?

_____

_____

_____

_____

What types of sights, scents, or sounds do you remember most from the dream?

_____

_____

_____

_____

What three things do you remember the most from the dream?

_____

_____

_____

_____

How would you interpret this dream in relation to your life and personality?

_____

_____

_____

_____

What was the overall emotion in the dream?

_____

_____

_____

_____

What do you think is the overall message?

_____

_____

_____

_____

What actions will you take in your daily life?

_____

_____

_____

_____

_____

_____

Draw the most memorable scene or symbol from your dream.

Dream

Date: ....

TYPE OF DREAM

* First-time Dream
* Scary Dream
* Happy Dream

* Recurring Dream
* Adventurous Dream
* Unique Dream

THEMES

* Driving
* Falling
* Flying
* Intimacy
* A Chase
* Trapped / Lost
* Failing

* Lateness
* Paralysis
* Searching
* Nudity
* Death
* Mirror
* School

How did this dream make you feel when you woke up?

_____

_____

_____

Description of the dream.

_____

_____

_____

_____

If this is a recurring dream, was there anything different that you can remember happened this time? If not, what common things do you always see in the dream?

_____

_____

_____

_____

What types of sights, scents, or sounds do you remember most from the dream?

_____

_____

_____

_____

What three things do you remember the most from the dream?

_____

_____

_____

_____

How would you interpret this dream in relation to your life and personality?

_____

_____

_____

_____

What was the overall emotion in the dream?

_____

_____

_____

_____

What do you think is the overall message?

_____

_____

_____

What actions will you take in your daily life?

_____

_____

_____

_____

_____

_____

Draw the most memorable scene or symbol from your dream.

Dream

Date: ....

TYPE OF DREAM

⭐ First-time Dream

⭐ Scary Dream

⭐ Happy Dream

⭐ Recurring Dream

⭐ Adventurous Dream

⭐ Unique Dream

THEMES

⭐ Driving

⭐ Falling

⭐ Flying

⭐ Intimacy

⭐ A Chase

⭐ Trapped / Lost

⭐ Failing

⭐ Lateness

⭐ Paralysis

⭐ Searching

⭐ Nudity

⭐ Death

⭐ Mirror

⭐ School

How did this dream make you feel when you woke up?

_____

_____

_____

Description of the dream.

_____

_____

_____

_____

_____

If this is a recurring dream, was there anything different that you can remember happened this time? If not, what common things do you always see in the dream?

_____

_____

_____

_____

What types of sights, scents, or sounds do you remember most from the dream?

_____

_____

_____

_____

What three things do you remember the most from the dream?

How would you interpret this dream in relation to your life and personality?

What was the overall emotion in the dream?

What do you think is the overall message?

What actions will you take in your daily life?

_____

_____

_____

_____

_____

_____

Draw the most memorable scene or symbol from your dream.

Dream

Date: ....

TYPE OF DREAM

★ First-time Dream   ★ Recurring Dream

★ Scary Dream   ★ Adventurous Dream

★ Happy Dream   ★ Unique Dream

THEMES

★ Driving   ★ Lateness

★ Falling   ★ Paralysis

★ Flying   ★ Searching

★ Intimacy   ★ Nudity

★ A Chase   ★ Death

★ Trapped / Lost   ★ Mirror

★ Failing   ★ School

How did this dream make you feel when you woke up?

_____

_____

_____

Description of the dream.

_____

_____

_____

_____

If this is a recurring dream, was there anything different that you can remember happened this time? If not, what common things do you always see in the dream?

_____

_____

_____

_____

What types of sights, scents, or sounds do you remember most from the dream?

_____

_____

_____

_____

What three things do you remember the most from the dream?

_____

_____

_____

_____

How would you interpret this dream in relation to your life and personality?

_____

_____

_____

_____

What was the overall emotion in the dream?

_____

_____

_____

_____

What do you think is the overall message?

_____

_____

_____

What actions will you take in your daily life?

_____

_____

_____

_____

_____

_____

Draw the most memorable scene or symbol from your dream.

Dream

Date: ....

TYPE OF DREAM

★ First-time Dream　　　　　★ Recurring Dream

★ Scary Dream　　　　　　　★ Adventurous Dream

★ Happy Dream　　　　　　　★ Unique Dream

THEMES

★ Driving　　　　　　　　　★ Lateness

★ Falling　　　　　　　　　★ Paralysis

★ Flying　　　　　　　　　　★ Searching

★ Intimacy　　　　　　　　　★ Nudity

★ A Chase　　　　　　　　　★ Death

★ Trapped / Lost　　　　　　★ Mirror

★ Failing　　　　　　　　　　★ School

How did this dream make you feel when you woke up?

_____

_____

_____

Description of the dream.

_____

_____

_____

_____

If this is a recurring dream, was there anything different that you can remember happened this time? If not, what common things do you always see in the dream?

_____

_____

_____

_____

What types of sights, scents, or sounds do you remember most from the dream?

_____

_____

_____

_____

What three things do you remember the most from the dream?

_____

_____

_____

_____

How would you interpret this dream in relation to your life and personality?

_____

_____

_____

_____

What was the overall emotion in the dream?

_____

_____

_____

_____

What do you think is the overall message?

_____

_____

_____

What actions will you take in your daily life?

_____

_____

_____

_____

_____

_____

Draw the most memorable scene or symbol from your dream.

Dream

Date: ....

TYPE OF DREAM

⭐ First-time Dream   ⭐ Recurring Dream

⭐ Scary Dream   ⭐ Adventurous Dream

⭐ Happy Dream   ⭐ Unique Dream

THEMES

⭐ Driving   ⭐ Lateness

⭐ Falling   ⭐ Paralysis

⭐ Flying   ⭐ Searching

⭐ Intimacy   ⭐ Nudity

⭐ A Chase   ⭐ Death

⭐ Trapped / Lost   ⭐ Mirror

⭐ Failing   ⭐ School

How did this dream make you feel when you woke up?

_____

_____

_____

Description of the dream.

_____

_____

_____

_____

_____

If this is a recurring dream, was there anything different that you can remember happened this time? If not, what common things do you always see in the dream?

_____

_____

_____

_____

What types of sights, scents, or sounds do you remember most from the dream?

_____

_____

_____

_____

What three things do you remember the most from the dream?

_____

_____

_____

_____

How would you interpret this dream in relation to your life and personality?

_____

_____

_____

_____

What was the overall emotion in the dream?

_____

_____

_____

_____

What do you think is the overall message?

_____

_____

_____

What actions will you take in your daily life?

_____

_____

_____

_____

_____

_____

Draw the most memorable scene or symbol from your dream.

Dream

Date: ....

TYPE OF DREAM

✴ First-time Dream   ✴ Recurring Dream

✴ Scary Dream   ✴ Adventurous Dream

✴ Happy Dream   ✴ Unique Dream

THEMES

✴ Driving   ✴ Lateness

✴ Falling   ✴ Paralysis

✴ Flying   ✴ Searching

✴ Intimacy   ✴ Nudity

✴ A Chase   ✴ Death

✴ Trapped / Lost   ✴ Mirror

✴ Failing   ✴ School

How did this dream make you feel when you woke up?

_____

_____

_____

Description of the dream.

_____

_____

_____

_____

_____

If this is a recurring dream, was there anything different that you can remember happened this time? If not, what common things do you always see in the dream?

_____

_____

_____

_____

_____

What types of sights, scents, or sounds do you remember most from the dream?

_____

_____

_____

_____

_____

What three things do you remember the most from the dream?

_____

_____

_____

_____

How would you interpret this dream in relation to your life and personality?

_____

_____

_____

_____

What was the overall emotion in the dream?

_____

_____

_____

_____

What do you think is the overall message?

_____

_____

_____

_____

What actions will you take in your daily life?

_____

_____

_____

_____

_____

_____

Draw the most memorable scene or symbol from your dream.

Dream

Date: ....

TYPE OF DREAM

★ First-time Dream ★ Recurring Dream

★ Scary Dream ★ Adventurous Dream

★ Happy Dream ★ Unique Dream

THEMES

★ Driving ★ Lateness

★ Falling ★ Paralysis

★ Flying ★ Searching

★ Intimacy ★ Nudity

★ A Chase ★ Death

★ Trapped / Lost ★ Mirror

★ Failing ★ School

How did this dream make you feel when you woke up?

_____

_____

_____

Description of the dream.

_____

_____

_____

_____

_____

If this is a recurring dream, was there anything different that you can remember happened this time? If not, what common things do you always see in the dream?

_____

_____

_____

_____

What types of sights, scents, or sounds do you remember most from the dream?

_____

_____

_____

_____

What three things do you remember the most from the dream?

_____

_____

_____

_____

How would you interpret this dream in relation to your life and personality?

_____

_____

_____

_____

What was the overall emotion in the dream?

_____

_____

_____

_____

What do you think is the overall message?

_____

_____

_____

What actions will you take in your daily life?

_____

_____

_____

_____

_____

_____

Draw the most memorable scene or symbol from your dream.

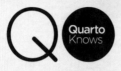

Inspiring | Educating | Creating | Entertaining

Brimming with creative inspiration, how-to projects, and useful information to enrich your everyday life, Quarto Knows is a favorite destination for those pursuing their interests and passions. Visit our site and dig deeper with our books into your area of interest: Quarto Creates, Quarto Cooks, Quarto Homes, Quarto Lives, Quarto Drives, Quarto Explores, Quarto Gifts, or Quarto Kids.

10 9 8 7 6 5 4 3 2

ISBN: 978-1-63106-820-1

Publisher: Rage Kindelsperger
Creative Director: Laura Drew
Managing Editor: Cara Donaldson
Senior Editor: Katharine Moore
Text: Leeann Moreau and Keyla Pizarro-Hernández
Illustrations: Sosha Davis

Printed in China

This book provides general information on various widely known and widely accepted self-care and wellness practices. However, it should not be relied upon as recommending or promoting any specific diagnosis or method of treatment for a particular condition, and it is not intended as a substitute for medical advice or for direct diagnosis and treatment of a medical condition by a qualified physician. Readers who have questions about a particular condition, possible treatments for that condition, or possible reactions from the condition or its treatment should consult a physician or other qualified healthcare professional.

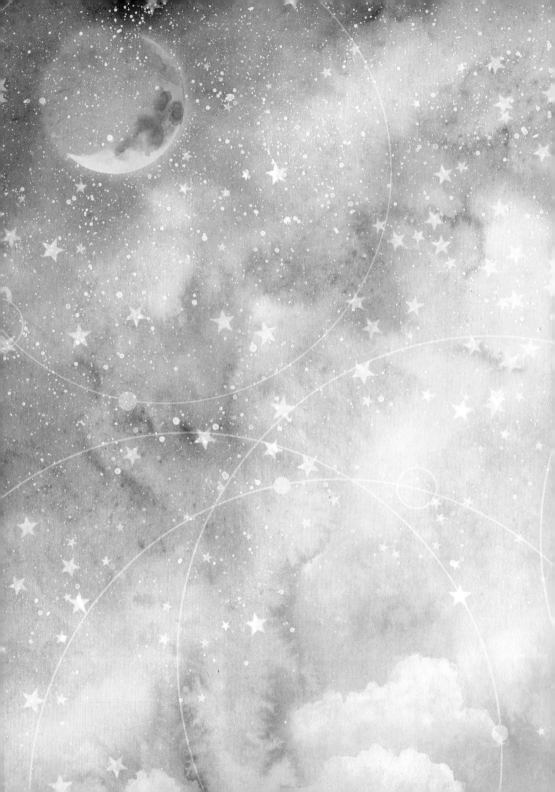